Sahar Elleuch
Kamel Kolsi

Anesthesia and preeclampsia

Sahar Elleuch
Kamel Kolsi

Anesthesia and preeclampsia

ScienciaScripts

Imprint

Cover image: www.ingimage.com

This book is a translation from the original published under ISBN 978-620-3-44252-6.

Publisher:
Sciencia Scripts
is a trademark of
Dodo Books Indian Ocean Ltd. and OmniScriptum S.R.L publishing group

120 High Road, East Finchley, London, N2 9ED, United Kingdom
Str. Armeneasca 28/1, office 1, Chisinau MD-2012, Republic of Moldova, Europe
Printed at: see last page
ISBN: 978-620-5-41923-6

Anaesthesia and pre-eclampsia

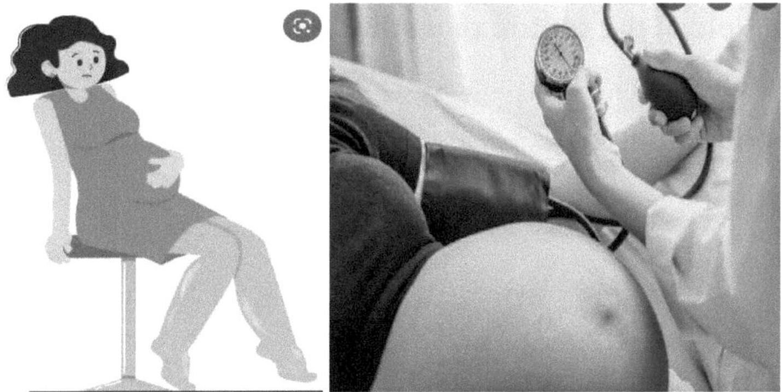

Author: Dr Sahar Elleuch

Contributor: Kamel Kolsi

Table of contents

Introduction

Introduction

Pre-eclampsia is a condition that occurs during pregnancy or post partum.

It is a very serious condition. It is one of the leading causes of maternal and neonatal mortality and morbidity in developing countries.

Approximately 10% to 15% of nulliparous women and 3% to 5% of multiparous women will develop gestational hypertension (GHT). Pre-eclampsia will occur in 3-7% of nulliparas and 1-3% of multiparas. [1]

The diagnosis of pre-eclampsia requires the presence of gravid hypertension associated with proteinuria (>0.3g/24H).

Severe pre-eclampsia is defined according to well-defined clinical and biological criteria.

Pregnancies that are complicated by severe pre-eclampsia are associated with particularly high perinatal morbidity and mortality.

Parturients with this condition must be hospitalised in facilities that allow for the care of the child, who is often premature or even very premature, and of the mother, who may present serious cardiovascular, neurological, renal and hepatic complications.

The main criteria for deciding whether or not to terminate a pregnancy depend on maternal and fetal conditions.

The objective of my work is to describe, through clinical observation, the perioperative management of a parturient suffering from severe pre-eclampsia while highlighting the role of the senior technician in this situation.

I. Clinical case study

I. Clinical case study:

I.1 Presentation of the woman in labour :

The study involved a 42 year old primiparous woman with a bi choriale bi amniotic twin pregnancy, at 34 weeks of amenorrhea +2 days, transferred from Medenine.

She was admitted to the intensive care unit for management of severe pre-eclampsia.

On the second day of hospitalisation, the pregnancy was complicated by fetal heart rhythm (FHR) abnormalities, and an emergency caesarean section was indicated.

I.2 Preoperative anaesthetic assessment :

I.2.1. Interrogation:

- Medical history :
  High blood pressure (on loxen + Dopanore)
- Surgical and anaesthetic history :
  Hysteroscopy with removal of a uterine polyp under anaesthesia (RA)
- Obstetrical history: Gestité: 01 (twin pregnancy)
  Parity: 02
  Abortion: 0
- Allergic history: No history of allergy
- Transfusion history: No history of transfusion
- Hematological history: No unusual bleeding
- Habits: No specific habits
  Passive smoking
- Current treatment: Loxen Lp 50mg 1cp*2/d
  Dopanore 250mg 2cp*3/d
  Enoxa preventive dose 0.4 1inj/d
  Mopral 40 1inj/d

I-2-2 Functional signs :

- **Cardiovascular:**

- Excellent stress tolerance: Met>7 (see appendix no:1)
- No chest pain or dyspnea

- **Respiratory:**

- Eupnea

- **Abdominal:**

- No abdominal or epigastric pain

- **Neurological:**

- Conscious, cooperative patient
- No headaches or visual disturbances

I-2-3 Clinical examination:

I-2-3-1 General :

- **Good general condition**
- Weight: 90 kg Height: 1.68 m
- Body mass index (BMI): 32 kg/m^2.
- Temperature: 37°C
- Normo-coloured Conjunctiva
- **Cardiovascular examination :**
  -Blood pressure (BP): 136/55 mm Hg
  -Pulse: 97 beats per minute (bpm)
  -Normal cardiac auscultation
  - Peripheral pulses present and symmetrical

- **Respiratory examination :**
  - Eupnea patient
  - Respiratory rate = 12 cycles/min
  -Hemoglobin oxygen saturation (SpO2) = 100%.

- Auscultation: No clear rales and vesicular murmurs

❖ **Abdominal examination :**

-Soft abdomen

-Abdominal tenderness

❖ **Neurological examination** :

-Cooperating conscious patient with GCS 15/15

- No sensory or motor deficit

❖ **Gynaecological examination :**

-No unusual bleeding

I-2-3-1 For anaesthetic purposes :

❖ Patient classified as ASA II (see Appendix 3)

❖ Tracheal intubation: expected to be difficult

- MALLAMPATI class: III
- Mouth opening > 35mm
- Thyro-chin distance > 65mm
- No dentures
- Good oral health
- No facial dysmorphia
- Good mobility of the spine

❖ Good venous capital

❖ Back examination: normal

I.2.4. Additional examinations :

❖ **Biological examination :**

- GS: B+ Rhesus: positive
- CBC: WBC: 6072mm^3 HB: 10g/dl Hte: 28% Platelets: 127 10^{3}mm^3
- ASAT: 23 UI ALAT: 10 UI
- Urea 5.3 mmol/L Creatine: 73 µmol/l
- TP: 96% TCA: 27/30 s
- BT: 19.3 µmol/L LDH: 190 IU/L
- 24-hour proteinuria: 0.42 g

❖ **Obstetrical ultrasound:**

- Twin 1: - hypotrophic PFE 1700g
  - Moderate oligohydramnios
  - Umbilical Doppler: 0.61
- Twin 2: - Eutrophic PFE 2300g
  -Normal amniotic fluid
  -Umbilical Doppler: 0.63

Information and consent of the patient:

The woman has been informed that she needs to be transferred to the operating theatre for an emergency caesarean section, and the procedure has been explained to her.

His consent was also obtained.

I.2.5. Preoperative instructions:

Reserve of 02 GCs + 10 PCs

Place in intensive care

I. 3 Intraoperative phase :

I.3.1 Preparation of the operating room :

As soon as I entered the room, I checked my checklist according to the A.P.A.V.O.I.R method

Suction equipment
✓ Operation of the suction source ✓ The connection ✓ Empty stop ✓ Suction probes of various sizes and suction hose
Infusion equipment
Catheters of different sizes (18G, 20G), clean compresses, antiseptic, tourniquet, plaster Physiological saline solution, infusion set with tap

Anaesthesia drugs and equipment for local anaesthesia
Sterile gloves, sterile compresses, sterile field, antiseptic, 25G rachi needle Plasters, 5ml syringe, 0.5mg ampoule of morphine ampoule of hyperbaric bupivacaine, ampoule of sufentanil, Prepared general anaesthesia drugs
Oxygenation and Ventilation Equipment
✓ The electricity connection ✓ Fresh gas connection (O2, NO2, air) ✓ Functional manual circuit (hose, bag, valve, mask, artificial nose) ✓ Functional mechanical circuit (hose, water trap, filter, capnograph) ✓ Unsaturated soda lime ✓ Functional bypass ✓ Pre-set alarm limits ✓ Adjustment of ventilation parameters ✓ Oxygen cylinder with a residual pressure of more than 50 bar
Intubation Tray
✓ Checked laryngoscope (handle, 2 different blades sizes 3 and 4) ✓ Sterile intubation probes of various sizes (6.5-7) ✓ Sterile GUEDEL cannulas ✓ Eichmann's Guide ✓ Magill clamp ✓ Plasters ✓ Stethoscope ✓ Syringe to inflate the balloon
Resuscitation drugs
✓ Emergency kit (Atropine, Ephedrine, Adrenaline and noradrenaline, Nicardipine, Lidocaine) ✓ Anaesthetic drugs ✓ Corticosteroids ✓ Furosemide ✓ Clonidine ✓ Functional defibrillator

Table 1:Operating room checklist

- **The different monitoring :**

-Electrocardioscope :

This monitoring system allows for continuous electrocardiogram (ECG) monitoring and includes 3 electrodes.

- Non-invasive pressure (NIP):

  - I have preset alarms for systolic and diastolic blood pressure.
  - Cuff sized to fit the patient's arm.

-Pulse oximeter :

I preset the alarms and checked the saturometer was working properly.

-Capnograph and gas analyser :

Setting alarms is essential.

I. 3.2 Anaesthesia procedure :

- Two anaesthesia technicians and one anaesthesiologist are present.
- On entering the room, the identity of the parturient was quickly checked.
- I checked the Mallampati class, the dental status, the mouth opening, the mobility of the cervical spine and the presence or absence of allergies.
- In addition, I checked the parturient's GS, the blood supply and the preoperative check-ups
- The parturient was placed on the operating table in DLG 15%.
- I have set up a monitoring system which consists of :
  - NIP
  - Scope with electrocardiogram with 3 leads
  - Saturometer
- The parameters collected :
  - BP: 136/55 mm hg
  - HR: 98 bp/min
  - Sp O2: 100%.
- I placed an 18 gauge venous line in the left upper limb.
- A 500cc saline filling was performed.

- The chosen anaesthetic technique: spinal anaesthesia.
- I administered 8mg of dexamethasone for the prevention of nausea and vomiting.

Preparation of materials :

The sterile equipment required for spinal anaesthesia includes:

- a spinal needle: a 25 gauge pencil point needle with an introducer

- a 5 ml syringe to collect the drugs

- a sterile field, sterile compresses, a cup for antiseptic and sterile gloves

- an occlusive bandage

- Anaesthetic drugs: Sufentanil (2cc = 10µg), Morphine (5ml=500µg), Bupivacaine 0.5% hyperbaric (4ml= 20mg)

Performing spinal anaesthesia :

- First, we explained the procedures to the patient and asked for her cooperation.
- The patient was positioned in a sitting position, with her chin tucked up to her chest, her "back rounded" with her forearms bent and her hands on her thighs.

  An aide helped her to maintain this position and to keep her shoulders and hips parallel.
- Afterwards, I did a first swabbing of the skin with an antiseptic.
- The anaesthetist put on sterile gloves and then applied a disinfectant (Betadine) in a spiral movement, going from the puncture point outwards without going back over the already treated area.
- Then he applied a sterile field to the whole back.
- He set up the introducer that allows the insertion of the spinal needle (25G) at the L4-L5 space.
- He then checked for cerebrospinal fluid reflux (clear CSF reflux) before fitting the syringe.
- Then he slowly injected a mixture of :
  - 100µg Morphine (1cc)
  - 2.5µg Sufentanil (or 0.5 cc)

- 10mg hyperbaric bupivacaine 0.5% (2cc)

- Finally, I applied a bandage.
- The parturient was positioned supine with her head elevated.
- I took the BP (122/99mmHg) and put the parturient on an oxygen monitor with 4l/min O2.
- Since the c-section is classified as a clean surgery, I administered 2g of augmentin as an antibiotic prophylaxis.
- The installation of the sympathetic block was marked by a fall in BP which was controlled by a simple filling.
- A sensory block: T4 was verified by light touch.
- An engine block with a bromide score of 2 was also checked
- In parallel, the surgical team prepared quickly.
- I started monitoring in the anaesthesia sheet (see appendix n°:4) SpO2, BP, HR every 2 min with the search for signs of pre-eclampsia (headache, visual disturbance, tinnitus, confusion...).
- The surgeon made a horizontal incision two fingers above the pubic bone (pfannenstiel incision)
- At the time of the hysterotomy, I make sure I have 100% oxygen.
- After clamping both cords and extracting both newborns, I administered 10 IU of syntocinon intravenously and 15 IU in the pouch to get a good uterine globe.
- Examination of the two newborns :
  - **1er twin**:

  Weight: 2.3kg

  Size: 50cm

  Head circumference: 35cm

  Gender: male

  Abgar's score: 8-9
  - **2éme twin** :

  Weight: 1.7kg

  Size: 46cm

  Head circumference: 34cm

  Gender: girl

  Abgar's score: 8-9
- Babies are transferred to the neonatal ward.

- After the artificial delivery, the surgeon sutured the uterus.
- To improve the tonicity of the uterine globe and following the surgeon's request, I added 10 IU of syntocinon in IV and 10 IU in the infusion (2nd bag)
- I monitored the patient until they were transferred to the post-op ward.

I.4. Post-operative phase :

In the ICU:

- Once I was transferred to the post-op ward, I passed on the necessary information to the nurse in charge.
  I monitored BP, pulse, diuresis, temperature, signs of pre-eclampsia (headache, visual disturbance, tinnitus, epigastric pain, confusion ...)
- I asked the parturient about the existence of nausea and vomiting.
- I looked for a bleed
- I calculated the BROMAGE score every 20min.
- The patient had no complications.
- The gynaecologist said that the uterine globe was good and that the bleeding was minimal.
- After ensuring HD stability, respiratory status, absence of motor block (Bromage score=0), I transferred the patient to the ward.

In the post partum ward :

At D1 post-op: 23/02/2020

- Apyretic patient
- Blood pressure profile :
  Systolic figures 110-150 mmHg, diastolic 70-60 mmHg Pulse: 92 Bpm
- Soft calves
- No signs of pre-eclampsia
- Transit restored and 1er lifted.
- She resumed her treatment: Dopanore 2cp*3/d, loxen 1cp*2/d
- Balance sheet :
  Hb: 9.7 g/dl
  Insert: 110,000 elts/mm^3.

TP: 98%.

At d2 post-op: 24/02/2020

- Apyretic patient
- Soft calves
- No signs of pre-eclampsia
- Blood pressure profile :
  Systolic figures range from 110 to 130 mmHg, diastolic from 60 to 70mmHg
  Pulse =92Bpm
- Control of TP and CRP, iono, NFS...
  Hb= 8.9 g/dl
  Plq: 145000 elts/mm^3
  TP=100% TCA= 26/29 s
  ASAT =19 UI ALAT= 6UI
  Urea= 3.9 mmol/ l creat=60 µmol/L
  24-hour proteinuria =0.3g/24H
- The patient had a hypokalaemia of 3.2mmol/L hence the administration of 3 ampoules in 500cc of saline for 3 hours with biological monitoring.
- The patient was put on loxen 1cp*2/d Dopanore 2cp*3/d and tardyferon 1cp*2/d

II. Discussion :

II. Discussion:

II. 1. Definitions:

*** Pregnancy-induced hypertension (PIH):**

PAS >140 mm Hg and/or DBP >90 mm Hg, occurring after 20 days' gestation and disappearing by the end of the 6th week postpartum [1].

*** Pre-eclampsia (PE)**

She associates with this HTAG a proteinuria at 300 mg/d or 2croix (test strips) [1].

*** Severe pre-eclampsia (SEP)**

Severe EP: EP with at least one of the following criteria:

- Severe hypertension (SAP > 160 mm Hg and/or DBP > 110 mm Hg)

- renal impairment with: oliguria (< 500 ml/24h) or creatinine > 135µmol/L, or proteinuria > 5 g/d

- Acute lung oedema or persistent epigastric bar or HELLP syndrome

- eclampsia or intractable neurological disorders (visual disturbances, polykinetic ROT, headache),

- thrombocytopenia < 100,000/mm³.

- Retroplacental haematoma (RPH) or fetal demise

HELLP syndrome: A combination of haemolysis, hepatic cytolysis and thrombocytopenia [2]

Eclampsia: occurrence of a tonic-clonic seizure in the context of hypertensive pathology of pregnancy. [2]

II.2 Epidemiology and risk factors:

In France, the frequency of pre-eclampsia is estimated to be between 1 and 3% in primiparous women, compared with 0.5 to 1.5% in multiparous women. [1]

In Tunisia, the frequency is 10 to 20% for primiparous women, compared with 3 to 5% for multiparous women. After a first pre-eclampsia, especially early and severe, there is a high risk of recurrence [1].

Six groups of factors can be identified: vascular, metabolic, immunological, genetic, placental and environmental factors such as [3] :

- Nulliparity, primipaternity
- Change of partner
- High maternal age
- Obesity
- Diabetes, Insolino resistance
- Chronic hypertension
- Chronic kidney disease
- Stress, work
- History of pregnancy complicated by PE or GVHD
- Long interval between two pregnancies, Pregnancy, multiple,
- Fetal congenital anomalies

II.3 Pathophysiology of the placenta in pre-eclampsia:

- Placental abnormality
- Decreased uteroplacental flow with placental ischaemic injury [1].
- Fetal impact: chronic suffering with dysharmonic intrauterine growth restriction (IUGR).
- Maternal impact: hypertension, thrombotic microangiopathy, coagulation disorders. [4]

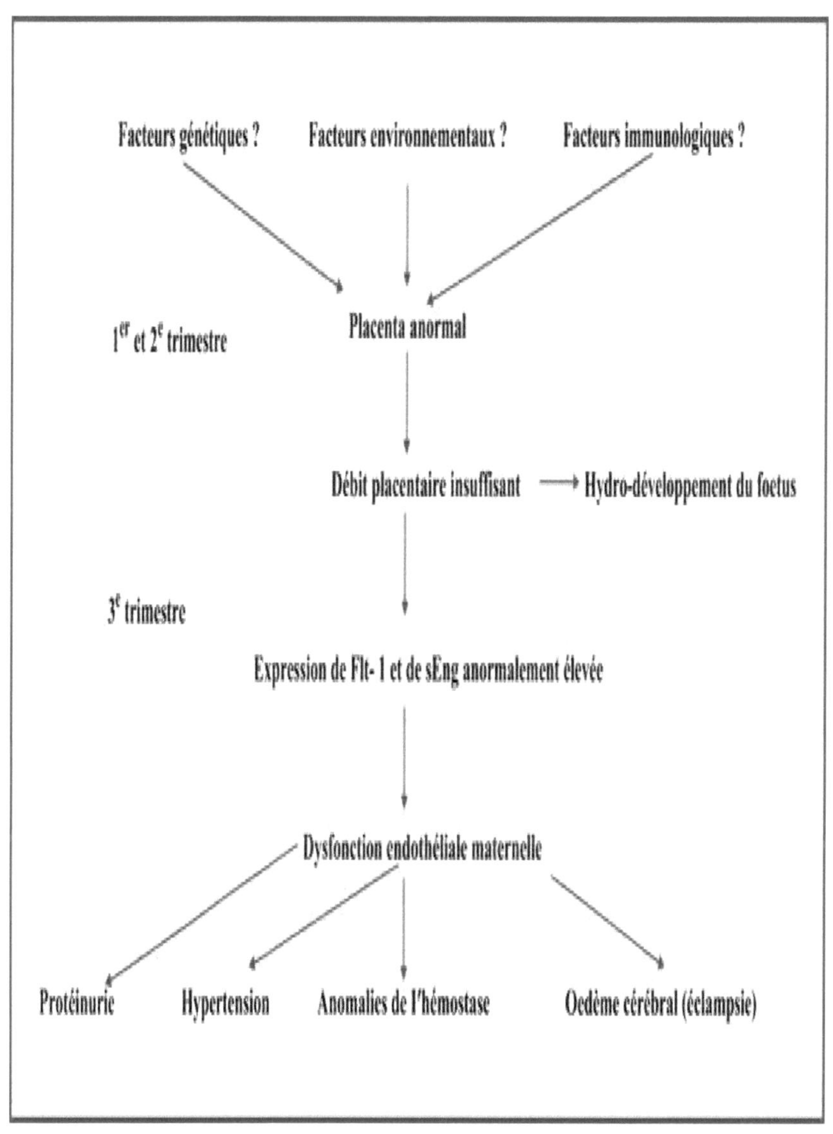

Figure 1Diagram summarising the mechanisms involved in the pathogenesis of pre-eclampsia

II. 4.Elements of surveillance for pre-eclampsia: [5]

II.4.1. Clinical assessment :

- The maternal state:

➤ **Blood pressure:**

The measurement of BP in pregnant women is difficult because of its variability.

➤ **Proteinuria on test strips :**

Massive proteinuria greater than or equal to 0.3g/d or 2 crosses on test strips.

➤ **Edema:**

When present, the oedemas are soft, white, diffuse, and cup-shaped. They extend beyond the declivity areas to the face, giving the appearance of a moon face.

➤ **Neurological signs** :

- Headaches
- confusion
- Sharp osteotendinous reflexes

➤ **Visual signs :**

Phosphenes, sensation of flying flies, decrease in visual acuity (retinal haemorrhage, papillary oedema)

➤ **Digestive signs:**

Are represented by: epigastric pain in bars, nausea, vomiting.

➤ **Serous effusion :**

In severe forms, particularly in the presence of oedema, ascites, pericardial effusions and pleural effusions have been described

- **Oliguria:** Is a sign of severity when it is < 20 ml/h.
- **Cardiac signs** :

Represented by chest pain, heart failure.

- **Bleeding signs** :
    - Petechial purpura
    - epistaxis
    - gingivorrhagia
- The fetal state:

On examination, the notion of a decrease in active fetal movements (AFM) and uterine height is sought.

Obstetrical examination for oligohydramnios or delayed IUGR

II.4.2. Biological assessment:

- maternal assessment:
- **Blood count - platelets :**
    - Severe or severe EP is defined as Thrombocytopenia< 100,000/mm3.
- **Hemolysis work-up :**
  Smear test for schizocytes
  Haptoglobin, LDH
  Free and Conjugated Bilirubin
- **Coagulation test :**

  PT, APTT, fibrinogen (DIC)

- **Renal assessment :**
  Blood ionogram, urea, creatinine, uricemia
- **Fasting blood glucose :**
- **Liver function tests:** AST/ALT, albumin, bilirubin, LDH
- **24-hour proteinuria:**
  Serious PE is defined as > 5g/ 24h
- **ECBU**

- **Fetal assessment:**
  - **Ultrasound:** biometry, vitality, amniotic fluid, umbilical and cerebral doppler
  - **Electrocardiotocogram:** signs of fetal distress

II. 5. Medical management of pre-eclampsia: [1]

The main decision criteria depend on maternal and fetal conditions .

Delivery and placental delivery are undoubtedly the definitive treatment for severe pre-eclampsia.

II. 5.1. Hospitalization criteria: [1]

- **As an outpatient** in cases of mild to moderate hypertension.
- **Maternal-fetal transfer** to a centre of appropriate level according to :
  -Gestational age of the child (if term <32SA)
  - the severity of severe pre-eclampsia and the possible need for maternal resuscitation.

II.5.2. Criteria for termination of pregnancy: [1]

- In the case of non-severe EP beyond 36 days' gestation, pregnancy termination should be considered.
- Severe EP beyond 34 weeks is an indication to terminate the pregnancy
- In the case of severe EP before 24 weeks' gestation, a medical termination of the pregnancy should be clearly discussed with the parents
- Indications for termination of pregnancy in severe EP between 24 and 34SAS can be maternal or fetal:

For maternal reasons :

- **Immediate:** Uncontrolled hypertension, eclampsia, acute pulmonary oedema (APO), retro placental haematoma (RPH), thrombocytopenia <50,000, sub capsular haematoma of the liver

- **After corticosteroid therapy for fetal maturation**
    - ✓ Rapidly worsening renal failure and/or persistent oliguria (< 100 ml / 4 hours) despite appropriate vascular filling
    - ✓ Persistent signs of impending eclampsia (headache or visual disturbances)
    - ✓ Persistent epigastric pain, progressive HELLP syndrome.

For fetal reasons :

- Repeated decelerations of the FCR
- Severe IUGR beyond 32 days' gestation,
- Reverse umbilical artery diastole, beyond 32 days' gestation

II. 5.3. Symptomatic treatment:

- **Position**

- Left lateral decubitus: promotes placental and renal perfusion

- **Antihypertensive:** If SAP > 160mmHg

Initial treatment: nicardipine: IV 1-4mg/h

Or labetalol bolus IV 1mg/kg

Maintenance: nicardipine: 1-4mg/h

Or labetalol IV: 5-20mg/h

Or clonidine: 15-40µg/h

- BP targets: SBP between 140 and 160mmHg and MAP between 100 and 120mmHg. [5]

Do not normalise the figures

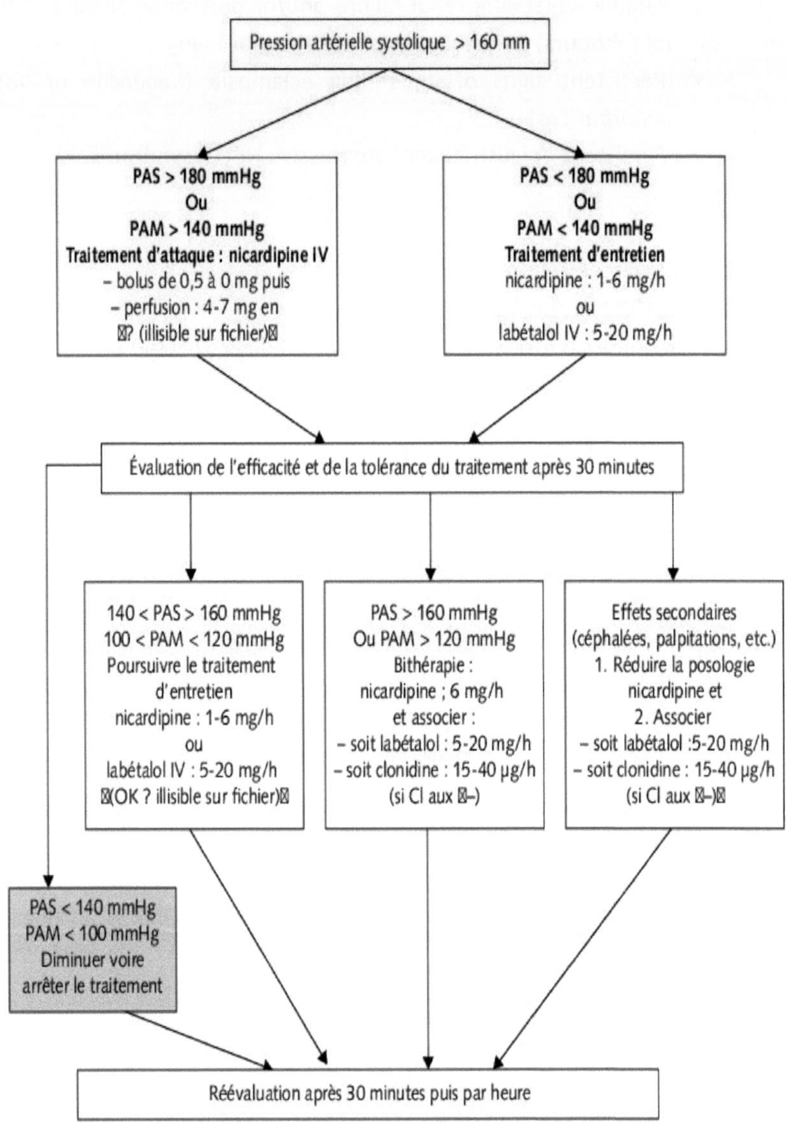

Figure 2Algorithm for prescribing antihypertensive treatment

- **Cautious volume expansion** if blood pressure falls on introduction of treatment [6].

- In cases of severe pre-eclampsia: prevention of eclampsia IV **magnesium sulphate** (4g bolus, then 1g/hr 3 days postpartum) is recommended in the presence of neurological signs (rebellious headaches, polykinetic ROT, visual disturbances) and in the absence of contraindication (renal insufficiency, neuromuscular diseases). [7]

II.5.4. Etiological treatment :

Termination of the pregnancy is the etiological treatment (medical termination of pregnancy or fetal extraction):

- In the case of non-severe EP beyond 36 days' gestation, pregnancy termination should be considered.
- Severe EP beyond 34 weeks is an indication to terminate the pregnancy
- In the case of severe EP before 24 weeks' gestation, a medical termination of the pregnancy should be clearly discussed with the parents

II.5.5 Associated measures:

-Antenatal corticosteroid therapy if extraction before 34 weeks' gestation. [8]

-Normalized sodium diet, rich in Ca and Mg

-Prevention of decubitus complications

II.6 Anaesthetic management :

The anaesthetic management of a pre-eclampsia PE patient should be guided by the following principles:

- ✓ The pre-anaesthetic assessment of the parturient, both clinically and biologically, should always be as close as possible to the procedure itself.
- ✓ Whatever anaesthetic technique is chosen, the aim should be to stabilise maternal blood pressure and avoid blood pressure peaks

II. 6.1. Preoperative phase:

II.6.1.1 Interrogation :

Full name, Age

Look for a possible history:
- Medical, surgical and obstetrical history

-Allergic, haematological, transfusion history

-List of medicines taken by the parturient.

II.6.1.2 Clinical examination:

General purpose :

- General condition of the woman in labour

-Weight, Height, BMI, Temperature

- Cardiovascular examination: BP, pulse, exercise tolerance, EMET, Lee score, dyspnoea, cardiac auscultation, etc.

- Respiratory examination: dyspnea, respiratory rate, cardiopulmonary auscultation, search for crepitus...

- Neurological examination: Glasgow score...

For anaesthetic purposes:

- Look for predictive factors for difficult intubation:

- History of difficult INT

- Search for VMD criteria

- OSA.

-The presence of macroglossia

- A mouth opening < 35mm and DTM < 60mm.

-MALLAMPATI III or IV.

- poor oral condition and presence of dentures

- lumbar spine stiffness

- Examination of the back
- Venous capital status

II.6.1.3 Para-clinical examination :

Biological examination: CBC with platelet count, GS, Rhesus

Liver function tests (GOT/GPT, bilirubin)

Haemostasis test (PT, TCK, fibrinogen)

Renal assessment: urea, creatinine - 24-hour proteinuria

Blood glucose, blood protein, blood urine.

Blood ionogram, ECBU, LDH ...

Obstetrical ultrasound

Chest X-ray: looking for PAO

Abdominal ultrasound: in case of HELLP syndrome to look for a sub capsular hematoma of the liver.

II.6.1.4. Consequences of pre-eclampsia:

Cardiovascular :

Severity of hypertension, signs of hypovolemia, oliguria, ...

Neurological: search for headaches, ROT vivacity, visual disturbances, presence of convulsions...

Abdominal: epigastric or right hypochondrium pain, constant abdominal pain associated with a "wooden uterus

Renal: Presence of oedema, Diuresis (ml/24 hours), Proteinuria

Haematological: Search for haemorrhages (epistaxis, conjunctival haemorrhage, gingivorrhage...)

Gynaecological: BCF, Haemorrhage

➡ **ASA classification**

➡ **Anaesthesia technique**

➡ **Information and consent of the patient**

Note: The Anaesthesia Consultation is most often performed in an emergency setting.

- After a pre-anaesthetic assessment of our parturient, she was classified as ASA II and an anaesthetic ok for spinal anaesthesia was made.

II.6.1.5 Preparation for anaesthesia :

In the majority of cases, the woman cannot be prepared because of the urgency and the short time allowed for the care.

- **Premedication :**

- Emergency caesarean sections cannot be pre-medicated due to the short time available
- Pregnant women are considered to have a full stomach, so the risk of pulmonary inhalation of gastric fluid is high.

- **Prophylaxis of regurgitation :**

- Prevention of gastric fluid inhalation is based on fasting status and control of gastric acidity by :
  - Ranitidine 150mg citrate at 0.3 molar
  - Tagamet citrate effervescent 200mg

- **Prophylaxis of thromboembolic disease**

- For our patient:

Premedication is not done because of the emergency. But as a prophylaxis for thromboembolic disease, she already had an injection of Enoxa 0.4 (1 day/24 hours) during the hospitalization in the intensive care unit.

II.6.1.6 Preparation of the operating room :

-Checklist for the operating room is done according to the A method. **P. A. V. O. I. R**

Suction

Infusion

Drugs and anaesthetic materials

Ventilation

Oxygenation

Intubation

Resuscitation drugs

Thus, monitoring equipment must be checked:

Electrocardioscope, NIBP, Pulse Oximeter, Capnograph and Gas Analyser...

II.6.2 Intraoperative phase:

Most women with severe pre-eclampsia deliver by caesarean section as a result of a worsening of the maternal clinical and biological condition and/or an alteration of the fetal condition. Depending on the urgency of the situation and the existence of haemostasis disorders, a choice is made between general and locoregional anaesthesia.

II.6.2.1. Choice of anaesthetic technique:

The choice of anaesthetic technique for caesarean section in the pre-eclamptic woman should be decided on a case-by-case basis depending on the patient, the impact of the anaesthetic technique on the newborn and the degree of urgency.

Classification of degree of urgency	Code Red	Code Orange	Code Green
Extraction	Less than 15 minutes or as soon as possible	Less than 30 minutes	Up to 60 minutes
Indications	Uterine rupture Procidence cord Fetal bradycardia >10 min without recovery Heavy bleeding DPPNI - eclampsia	Forceps failure Significant abnormalities of the FHR	Stagnation Dystocia Trigger failure
Types of anaesthesia	GA or "Epidural extension" (if local organisation optimised and if injection on call in APD)	Epidural extension Spinal anaesthesia	Epidural extension Spinal anaesthesia

Table 2Classification of degree of urgency

ALR is preferred [2] in the absence of contraindications to prevent the risks of GA such as difficult IOT, inhalation, hypertensive surge with classical rapid induction: stroke, OAP, drug interactions.

- For our clinical case, the anaesthetist chose spinal anaesthesia for several reasons:
  - degree of urgency: code orange (Significant FHR abnormalities) from which spinal anaesthesia is recommended.
  - Stomach full due to emergency and pregnancy hence risk of inhalation
  - presence of difficult intubation criteria
  - no contraindication to spinal anaesthesia

II.6.2.2. Spinal anaesthesia:

❖ The benefits:

- easy and simple to implement
- Preventing the risk of inhalation and difficult intubation
- Avoiding the baby's exposure to anaesthetics
- To enable the woman in labour to be conscious at the time of her baby's birth.
- Prevent hypertensive flare-ups at the time of laryngoscopy and extubation.
- Reducing postoperative pain
- Reduce the postoperative consequences induced by general anaesthesia (less drowsiness, less sore throat...)
- Enable easy clinical monitoring of the condition of the parturient through questioning

❖ The disadvantages

- Complete failure or laterality
- Risk of voltage drop
- Risk of extension of the engine block
- AR cannot cover eclampsia and altered consciousness
- Nausea and vomiting
- Shivers-Hypothermia

Local anaesthetics and anaesthetic drugs for spinal anaesthesia:

Ropivacaine, bupivacaine and levobupivacaine are the only local anaesthetics with marketing authorisation for intrathecal injection.

Lidocaine 5% is no longer approved for this indication due to the risk of transient root irritation syndrome and cauda equina syndrome.

For a caesarean section the use of bupivacaine is the best choice [9].

Bupivacaine 0.5% hyperbaric :

- Dose 8 to 12 mg (1cc=5mg) presentation 4cc=20mg
- Sensory block is achieved after 5 to 20 minutes at the most. The duration of the sensory and motor block is 2 to 2.5 hours.
- Injection of excessive amounts of bupivacaine into the cerebrospinal fluid and/or failure to maintain position after spinal anaesthesia is likely

to result in extension of the block which may lead to total spinal anaesthesia and neurological and cardiac toxicity [10].

- The lower the dose: [10]
  - the level of the sensory block is lower
  - the engine block is less intense.
  - the duration of the block is shorter
- Below 6 mg no engine block
- For 8 mg the incidence of the engine block is 53%.

Fat-soluble morphines: sufentanil or fentanyl are recommended in combination with bupivacaine to provide better intraoperative comfort and longer duration of analgesia.

Sufentanil :

- Sufentanil is the morphine of choice [11].
- Recommended doses are 2.5-5 µg sufentanil
- Short onset of action a few minutes - Duration of action 2 to 3 hours
- allows the necessary dose of local anaesthetics to be reduced, which in turn allows the intensity of the sympathetic block and motor block to be attenuated.
- Less risk of respiratory depression than Morphine
- Improved quality of analgesia without prolonging the duration of the block
- Effective analgesia with low doses AL
- Longer acting than fentanyl
- Low nausea, low pruritus

Fentanyl :

- The recommended doses are 10-25 µg

- Reduces the dose of local anaesthetics required with effective analgesia [12].
- Reduced block installation time
- Less pain and reduced nausea and vomiting during surgery
- Does not reduce the postoperative effectiveness of perimedullary morphine

morphine :

- At a dose of 0.1 to 0.2 mg
- A prolonged duration of action (4-7 h) allows postoperative analgesia to be covered [12].
- a risk of respiratory depression, pruritus and urinary retention
- The use of morphine allowed a reduction in postoperative morphine consumption (24 hours).

- In our clinical case we used the minimum effective doses to have a satisfactory spinal anaesthesia that covers the whole time of surgery with :
    - 10 mg hyperbaric bupivacaine 0.5% (1cc=5mg): effective dose to achieve the desired level of anaesthesia with minimal risk of failure and adverse effects.
    - 2.5µg sufentanil (1cc=5µg): the fat-soluble morphine of choice with a short onset of action and long duration of action. It improves the quality of analgesia without prolonging the duration of the block
    - 100µg Morphine (1cc=100µg): With this dose the risk of respiratory depression is low. A higher dose does not provide better postoperative analgesia, but does increase the risk of nausea and pruritus.

- **Spinal anaesthesia:**

- The woman is seated in a sitting position, with her chin towards the father, her back rounded, her forearms bent and her hands on her thighs.

- Locating the puncture site (the space easiest to puncture is chosen between L3-L4 and L4-L5). The contours of the spinous processes and a horizontal line passing between the two anterior superior iliac spines are drawn [9] (figure 2). [9] (Figure 2).

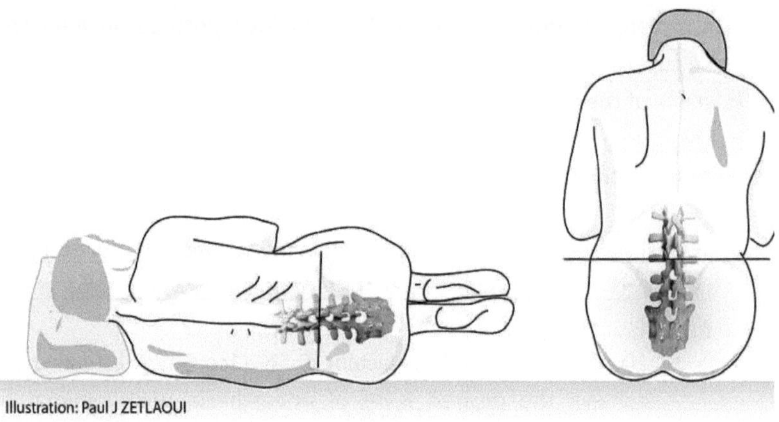

Figure 3Locating the puncture site

- Brush and apply sterile drapes over the entire back sterilely
- Placement of the introducer which allows the insertion of the spinal needle in the L3-L4 or L4-L5 space.
- check for reflux of a drop of clear CSF before fitting the syringe containing the anaesthetic products.

- Slowly inject the mixture of local anaesthetic and anaesthetic drugs (1 ml every 3 seconds). During the injection, the needle should be kept still with verification of the correct position of the needle by aspirating CSF before and during the injection.

- Performing a dressing

- place the woman in the supine position with her head elevated

- Monitoring the installation of the sensory block

- assess the motor block by bending the knees and toes

Intraoperative monitoring parameters in spinal anaesthesia:

Intraoperative monitoring is always systematic and consists of

- monitoring of vital parameters: BP, Pulse, SpO2 ...
- monitoring of diuresis
- monitoring the quality of analgesia.
- clinical monitoring: vagal discomfort, allergic reaction, nausea and vomiting...
- Toxicity monitoring of local anaesthetics: Atrioventricular conduction disorders, cardiac arrest, convulsion, coma...

- in the case of our parturient: monitoring of vital parameters (BP, Pulse, Diuresis, SpO2..), clinical monitoring, search for signs of PE. (see appendix n°:4)

II.6.2.3. Combined peri-spinal anaesthesia (CRP): [14]

The benefits of CRP over AR for Caesarean section in a woman with pre-eclampsia have not been demonstrated. Performing CRP for caesarean section in the pre-eclampsia woman provides a haemodynamic profile comparable to that obtained with epidural anaesthesia.

II.6.2.4. Epidural anaesthesia (APD) :

When a catheter has already been placed for analgesia during labour, extraction of the epidural for caesarean section is possible, by injecting 15-20 ml of 2% adrenalin lidocaine + 5-10µg sufentanyl

APDL and AR have a comparable effect on haemodynamic stability.

II.6.2.5. Contraindication to ALR: [14]

The absolute contraindications are:

- uncorrected hypovolaemia
- coagulation disorders
- sepsis at the puncture site
- the patient's refusal.
- Retro placental haematoma
- Treatment with aspirin + anticoagulant
- Eclampsia
- Acute fetal distress (extraction<5 min)

The relative contraindications are:

- neurological deficit, migraine and spinal cord disease,
- a febrile syndrome,
- spinal deformities, history of sciatica or low back pain

II.6.2.5. General anaesthesia:

General anaesthesia is most often used because of the frequency of coagulopathy and the extreme urgency.

- **Benefits:**

The advantages of general anaesthesia are its speed, reliability and safety in terms of respiratory and neurological safety, especially if there is pulmonary oedema, altered consciousness or even recurrent convulsions. Intraoperative monitoring of SpO2 and partial end-tidal pressure of CO2 (PETCO2) is important.

- **Disadvantages:**

The disadvantages of general anaesthesia remain significant. Frequent severe hypertensive attacks put the patient at risk of cerebral haemorrhage or left ventricular failure with pulmonary oedema. Emergency antihypertensive drugs should be ready during anaesthetic induction.

Remifentanyl is used at a dose of 1µg/kg at induction in pre-eclampsia to limit intubation-related hypertensive spikes

The risk of inhalation of digestive fluid is increased by tracheal intubation, which is often difficult (pharyngo-laryngeal oedema, bleeding from fragile mucous membranes). The material necessary to overcome an intubation difficulty must be prepared in the operating room.

- **Course of the general anaesthesia :**

Installation and pre-oxygenation:

- The installation of the parturient has three specific features
  - ✓ prevention of cave syndrome by a cushion under the right buttock or a marked left-hand tilt of the table
  - ✓ prevention of gas embolism during delivery by a slight proclivity
  - ✓ prevention of nerve compression due to posture, which is common in nerve tissue sensitised by pregnancy.
- Monitoring
- Two large-calibre peripheral venous lines are put in place.
- Prevention of gastric fluid inhalation is based on fasting and control of gastric acidity with Ranitidine 150mg citrate 0.3 molar
- Pre-oxygenation is carried out in a semi-seated position for 3 to 4 min with spontaneous ventilation with fiO2=100% and with fresh gas flow (≥ 10 l/min)
- When the fraction of tele-expiratory oxygen (FeO2) > 90%, pre-oxygenation is considered effective.

Induction sequence :

Modified quick sequence

Morphine drugs :

The addition of a morphine is classically recommended in women with EP from induction, not after cord clamping, as it limits hypertensive surges

Alfentanil :

- At a dose of (10µg/kg)
- Its effects on the foetus are moderate.
- It should be injected 2 minutes before induction to be effective on maternal haemodynamics.

Remifentanil :

- 0.5 to 1 µg/kg at induction then 0.15 to 0.2 µg/kg/min (stop 1 min before fetal extraction)
- the morphine of choice but cases of neonatal respiratory depression have been described and are of very limited duration

Narcotics :

Thiopental and propofol are two anaesthetic agents of choice.

Thiopental :

- the doses used in pregnant women are 35% lower than those used outside of pregnancy
- The onset of action is 20-40 seconds, the maximum effect is reached in 60 seconds and the duration of action is 5 minutes.
- During induction in the mother, thiopental increases heart rate (+20%), blood pressure (+15-30%) and uterine artery resistance, thus decreasing uteroplacental blood flow. These changes disappear as soon as the patient is intubated.
- At the usual doses (4-5 mg/kg) during general anaesthesia, there is no decrease in Apgar score compared to locoregional anaesthesia.

Propofol :

- Induction with propofol is identical to that with thiopental at the doses usually used in obstetrics.
- Propofol rapidly crosses the placental barrier
- When the dose is less than 2-2.5 mg/kg, there are no changes in the Apgar score in the baby

Curares :

Succinylcholine :

it is recommended for :

- Preferably to ensure rapid induction and intubation when Succinylcholine is not contraindicated:
  - hyperkalemia
  - Allergy to this product or to a non-depolarising curare (
  - Personal or family history of neuromuscular disease (malignant hyperthermia, myopathy, paraplegia, etc.)

- If there is a contraindication to succinylcholine, Rocuronium (1 to 1.2mg/kg) is used.

Orotracheal intubation:

- Given the physiological changes during pregnancy, intubation of pregnant women is 8 times more difficult, especially in cases of severe PE due to the mucosal oedema significantly affecting the Cormack.
- Intubation is performed with the Sellick manoeuvre maintained.
- The Sellick manoeuvre involves manual occlusion of the oesophagus at the cervical level by firmly compressing the cricoid cartilage on the cervical vertebrae while general anaesthesia is induced.
- This manoeuvre is carried out in the absence of contraindications:

  - ✓ Active vomiting
  - ✓ Cervical spine injuries
  - ✓ Laryngeal trauma
  - ✓ Tracheostomy Pharyngeal diverticulum
  - ✓ Foreign body in the airway
  - ✓ Cervical spinal cord injury

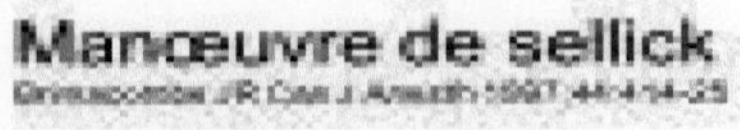

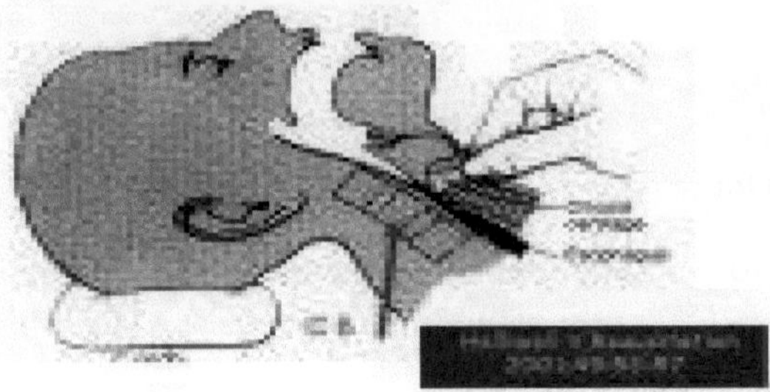

Figure 4:Sellick manoeuvre

Maintenance of anaesthesia :

- Maintenance is done with a halogen or a narcotic:
- NO2 passage is low. Prolonged administration increases the risk of neonatal depression
- Propofol can be used for maintenance with a dose of <9mg/kg/min.
- Curare is not always necessary, especially if the extraction is brief
- After fetal extraction, maintenance is maintained with either halogen or propofol by electric syringe
- Morphinics: Fentanyl, sufentanil, remifentanil
- Oxytocin allows good uterine retraction after delivery and a good uterine globe (Maximum dose 40 IU)
- Antibiotic prophylaxis is most often carried out after clamping the cord. Some teams recommend its administration before the incision (2G Augmentin).

II.6.3. Post-operative phase :

II.6.3.1. In case of ALR :

Post-operative monitoring: The patient is monitored in the recovery room or in the operating theatre until the sensory and motor blocks have completely disappeared.

- <u>For our parturient:</u> postoperative monitoring of BP, HR, SpO2, diuresis, nausea and vomiting, search for signs of PE, calculation of Bromage Score... (see appendix n°:5)

II.6.3.2. In case of GA :

The awakening is a critical period, which is accompanied by some significant risks.

Signs of awakening :

- Hemodynamics: HR, BP
- Respiratory: resumption of spontaneous ventilation
- Neuromotricity: Eye opening, responses to simple commands, +/-test for curarization
- Antagonistation :
    - Only curares with anticholinergics: 40µg/kg Prostigmine combined with 20µg/kg Atropine
- Oral-pharyngeal and tracheal aspirations

Extubation :

Extubation criteria :

- **Respiratory:** no cyanosis, symmetrical and regular breathing, no draught and FR between 12 and 20 cycles per min
- **Neurological:** oriented reaction, eye opening on simple command, no neurological deficit
- **Cardiovascular:** BP and HR within 20-30% of baseline
- **Neuromuscular**: raise head more than 5 seconds, shake hands, stick out tongue, possibility of swallowing, no shivering with Temperature>36.5°C
- Absence of complications
- Table top recovery or transfer of the intubated patient to the ICU

Analgesia: After general anaesthesia, analgesia is managed by a combination of drugs: morphine (2 to 3 mg), NSAIDs and paracetamol, which provide satisfactory pain relief. Self-controlled intravenous administration of morphine gives better results than the intravenous route. [13]

II.7. Complications :

II.7.1. Complications related to general anaesthesia :

- Traumatic intubation: dental injuries, sore throat, difficulty swallowing.
- prolonged position on the operating table resulting in compressions
- nerve, muscle and skin disorders
- Memory problems, reduced ability to concentrate
- Wake-up delay
- Nausea, vomiting
- Anaphylactic shock/ Allergy
- Hypertensive peak at the time of intubation and extubation

II.7.2 Complications related to locoregional anaesthesia :

	Complications	Treatments
During the puncture	vagal discomfort	ephedrine atropine
At the installation of the block	hypotension bradycardia drowsiness confusion convulsion nausea vomiting dyspnea apnea	ephedrine filling atropine ephedrine filling anticonvulsant in case of convulsion dexamethasone oxygen ventilation sedation
Late complications	urinary retention	urinary catheter

	headaches	
	cranial pair paralysis	analgesic supine position
	traumatic nerve root damage	
	other neurological complications: haematoma, sepsis	neurologist's opinion
	Toxicities of local anaesthetics: Neurological and cardiac	Oxygenation, hypnovel after cord clamping

Table 3Incidents and accidents: therapeutic management

II.7.3 Complications of pre-eclampsia:

-Eclampsia

- HELLP syndrome

- Retro placental haematoma

-Kidney damage

-Fetal complications:

- growth retardation during pregnancy
- prematurity, sometimes extreme, and its potential consequences
- death in 2-5% of cases

III. Role of the senior anaesthesia technician :

III. Role of the senior anaesthesia technician :

Pre-operative phase:

- Check the operating room checklist and prepare it for the reception of the woman in labour
- Maintain and check daily, by means of the corresponding list recommended by SFAR, the state of operation and sterilisation of equipment (circuits, respirators, monitoring)
- Take charge of the patient, check her identity, verify the planned operation and the site to be operated on, monitor and supervise the patient
- Reassure the patient and ensure her physical and psychological comfort

Intraoperative phase:

- Work in collaboration with the anaesthetist in the practice of anaesthesia
- Monitor and maintain the anaesthesia and notify the doctor of any abnormalities
- Monitor and control signs of pre-eclampsia
- Prevent, detect and treat complications of anaesthesia
- Ensure good haemodynamic and respiratory monitoring, in particular the position of the intubation tube, capnia.

Post-operative phase:

- Participate in the revival period and judge the quality and criteria of revival
- Accompany the woman to the ICU and ensure that information is passed on to the staff.
- Continuous monitoring of the procedure, maintaining the patient's respiratory autonomy, circulatory balance and neurological recovery.
- Monitoring for signs of pre-eclampsia
- Initiating, anticipating and optimising the management of postoperative pain
- To detect complications directly linked to the surgical act, and requiring the advice of the operator, often urgently (haemorrhage, neurological deficit, respiratory distress attributable to the surgical act)

- When faced with an emergency, carry out actions within his/her competence according to an established protocol.

Conclusion

Conclusion:

Pre-eclampsia remains one of the main causes of maternal and foetal mortality in the world. It combines gravidic hypertension and proteinuria >0.3g/24H, revealing itself from the 20th week of amenorrhea.

This is a multi-visceral condition where the only treatment is termination of pregnancy and placental delivery.

Caesarean delivery remains the most common indication for women with pre-eclampsia due to maternal and/or fetal condition.

The anaesthetic management of a patient with pre-eclampsia during caesarean section varies from case to case. It may be general anaesthesia or LRA, subject to contraindications and urgency, but LRA should be preferred.

The role of the anaesthesia technician is essential in the management of a pre-eclamptic woman during the pre-, intra- and postoperative stages. This management requires multidisciplinary collaboration with the anaesthetist and the surgical team.

Prevention of pre-eclampsia requires good antenatal care.

Bibliography

Bibliography :

[1] Pottecher T, Luton D, Zupan V, et al, Multidisciplinary management of severe pre-eclampsia , 2009, 22;11-21

[2] Pottecher T, Resuscitation of severe pre-eclampsia, Expert Conference, 2009, 2-84299-235

[3] 2002Pottecher T. J Gynecol Obstet Reprod 2001; 30: 121

[4] Chaoui A, Tyane M, Belouali R, Prise en charge de la pré éclampsie et de l'éclampsie. 2nd national consensus conference MOROCCO, 19-20-21

[5] Sibai BM, Dekker G, Kupfermine M. Pre-eclampsia, 2005; 365: 785-99

[6] M Brel, L Dubios-Gozlan, P.Dailland et al, Protocoles d'anesthésie réanimation obsétrical ,2011

[7] Moignet C, Diemunsch P, PottecherT. Intensive care anaesthesia and pre-eclampsia. Conférences d'actualisation. 2003 : 387-406

[8] Isler C.M., Barrilleaux P.S., Rinehart B.et al. Postpartum seizure prophylaxis: using maternal clinical parameters to guide therapy. Obstet Gynecol 2003; 101: 66-9

[9] Edouard D. Hypertension and pre-eclampsia. In: Anesthésie-Réanimation Obstétricale. Paris, 2009: 179-93.

[10] Arzola C, Wieczorek PM. Efficacy of low-dose bupivacaine in spinal anaesthesia for Caesarean delivery. 2011;107:308-18

[11] Yves Auroy, Guy Aya, Françoise Bayoumeu et al. Perimedullary blocks in adults. 2007 -720-752

[12] ZOUMENOU E. Les Agents de la rachianesthésie : efficacité et effets secondaires Janvier 2000 - 324-321

[13] Ginosar Y, Mirikatani E, Drover D, et al. intrathecal hyperbaric bupivacaine coadministered with opioids for cesarean delivery. Anesthesiology 2004;100:676-82

[14] Palmer CM, Nogami WM, Van Maren G, et al. Postcesarean epidural morphine 2000; *90*: 887-91.

[15] ELEDJAM JJ., BRUELLE P., CUVILLON P. Contraindications to spinal anaesthesia in adults. 40th Congress of Anesthesia and Intensive Care 1998 220-67

Annexes

CONSULTATION PRÉ-ANESTHÉSIQUE

DATE 22/02/2020 **DOCTEUR** (Cachet) Rdte Jáafar

☐1 A distance (c.externe) ☐ 2 Non à distance ☐ 3 Visite préop ou au bloc

Diagnostic chirurgical : C/s pour anomalies de RCF **N° D chir :** ....

Intervention envisagée : Césarienne **Prévue le :** ....

☐ 1 Programmée ☐ 2 Urgence diférée ☒ 3 Urgence

ATCDS Chirurgicaux / Anesthésiques :

- Hysteroscopie + exerese d'un polype utérin ss RA

ATCDS Médicaux / Obstétricaux : G I P II A 0

- chiffres tensionnelle elevé : ss (Loxen + Dopamine)
- Ygemellaire TAG - 34 SA + 03J

Tolérance à l'effort (☐angor et / ou ☐ dyspnée) : ∅

☐1 : Excellente (>7 MET): ☐2 : modérée (4-7 MET) ; ☐3 : mauvaise (<4 MET)

ALLERGIE : ☐1 oui .... ☒ 2 non

Saignement inhabituel : ☐1 oui .... ☒ 2 non

Myopathie familiale : ☐1 oui .... ☒ 2 non

Tabac : ☐1oui (☐ actuel (.....PA) ☐ severé (.....PA) ☒ Passif ☐ 2 non

TRANSFUSIONS ANTÉRIEURES/ DATES :

∅

TRAITEMENT EN COURS :

- Loxen
- Dopamine
- Enoxa dose preventive 0,4 1inj /j
- Mopral 40 1inj /j

EXAMEN CLINIQUE :

Poids : ....90...... Kg ; Taille : ....cm ; **BMI** ....

Etat général : ☒ 1 : Bon ; ☐ 2 : moyen , ☐ 3 : mauvais

Capital veineux : ☒ 1 : Bon ; ☐ 2 : moyen , ☐ 3 : mauvais

Auscultation cardio pul : ☒ 1 : Normale ☐ 2 : Non (..........................)

Examen du dos : ☒ 1 : Normale ☐ 2 : Non (..........................)

TA = 136 / 55 mmHg Pouls = 97 bpm Spo_2 à l'air ambiant = 98 %

Annex No. 1

INTUBATION TRACHEALE ☐ 1 facile ☒ 2 difficile

Classe de MALLAMPATI : [I] [II] [III] (circled) [IV]

Ouverture buccale : ☐ < 35 mm ☒ > 35 mm

Distance thyro-mentonière ☐ < 65 mm ☒ > 65 mm

☐ Dysmorphie faciale ☐ Mauvaise mobilité du rachis cervical

☐ Prothése dentaire ☐ Mauvaise état bucco-dentaire Ø

EXAMENS BIOLOGIQUES (date: 20/02/2020..............)

☐ **GS** B+ ☐ **Rhésus** positif ☐ **Phénotype**

☐ **RAI :** .... date : ....

☐ **NFS : GB** 6,72 Elts/mm³ **Hb**...10......g/dl **Hte**...28...............%

☐ **Plaquettes** : 127 ....10^3 ☐ **TP**.............. % ☐ **TCA :**..................

☐ **Glycémie** .... ☐ **Urée:**.................... ☐ **Créatinémie** ...73 µmol/L...

☐ **Natrémie** .... ☐ **Kaliémie**........ ☐ **Chlorémie** .... ☐ **RA**............

RADIO THORAX : Coeur ☐ **V1** ☐ **V2** ☐ **V3**

Anomalies parenchyme ☐ **oui** .... ☐ **Non**

ECG : Déviation axiale ☐ **oui** .... ☐ **Non**

Tr du Rythme ☐ **oui** .... ☐ **Non**

Tr repolarisation ☐ **oui** .... ☐ **Non**

Tr conduction ☐ **oui** .... ☐ **Non**

Commentaires : ....

AUTRES EXPLORATIONS :

Annex 2

CONCLUSION ET CONSIGNES PRE- OPÉRATOIRES

OK POUR L 'ANESTHÉSIE ☒ OUI (sous reserve des récommandations) ☐ NON

CLASSE ASA: ☐ ASA 1 ☒ ASA 2 ☐ ASA3 ☐ ASA4 ☐ ASA5

TYPE D 'ANESTHÉSIE PRÉVU:

☐ Anesthésie Générale:(drogues ___)

☐ Estomac plein ☐ Intubation trachéale prévue difficile)

☒ Anesthésie ou/et analgésie loco régionale :(R A)

☐ Consentement (Patient ou tuteur) : ☐ OUI ☐ NON

PLACE EN RÉANIMATION EN POST OPÉRATOIRE ☐ OUI ☐ NON

ANBULATOIRE / ☐ OUI ☒ NON

EXAMENS/ AVIS à FAIRE : ☐ OUI (___) ☐ NON

COMMANDE DE SANG ET DÉRIVÉS :

☐ FERME (___)

☐ RESERVE (___)

☐ NON

TRAITEMENT À ARRETER : ___

PREMEDICATION : ___

VISITE PRE-OPÉRATOIRE

Date : __/__/__

Docteur : ___ Signature : ___

Consignes particulières: ___

Annex No. 3

Annex No:4

SURVEILLANCE EN SALLE DE RÉVEIL

Date : 22/02/2020. Infirmier : ....

T réel	T0	T20	T40	T60	T80	T100	T120	T140	T160	T180
FC/mn	78	75	74	78	83					
PAS	117	121	142	156	138					
PAD	69	77	68	92	97					
PAM	90	93	95	115	115					
SpO2	98%	98%	98%	98%	99%					
FResp/mn										
diurèse	600cc				1250					
Température					jdi					
pertes sanguines 0 +++	–	–	–	–	–					
EVA ou OPS ou Cheops										
Score sédation S De 1 à 4										
Nausée N ou Vomiss V	+/-	-/-	-/-	-/-	-/-					
Score ALDRETE										
Score de BROMAGE	3	2	0	0	0					
Perfusion	SSI	8mg dexaméthasone + 80mg Tagamet								
Antalgiques		+ 10mg primpéran.								
	Bilan	XX								

T0 entrée en salle de réveil (noter l'heure) : 3...h ...35.......mn

Décision de sortie de la salle de réveil : Heure .6h50 Anesthésie .Pr. Jaafar

Annex No. 5

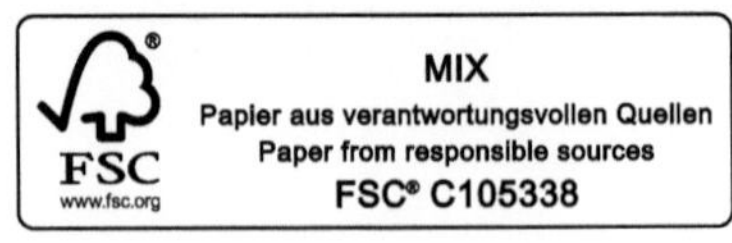

Printed by Books on Demand GmbH, Norderstedt / Germany